Natural Homemade Recipes for Long Healthy Hair

Organic, Simple & Do it Yourself Recipes for Perfect Hair

Disclaimer

How this eBook is Just for Your Hair!

Hair is thought to be the core of beauty for both men and women, but it has always held more significance for women. Women who have long, silky hair are considered to be luckier and become an icon of envy for many. Some have it naturally, while others work to improve their hair condition. In these times and atmospheric conditions, keeping your hair healthy and beautiful is not only difficult, it is very time consuming too. But that is not the only difficulty. Another issue with the rising economy is the exorbitant amounts of money you have to spend to even buy something as simple as shampoo! Long, healthy hair has become a coveted dream for most women.

This is the exact reason why this eBook has been written so that you can find everything you need to know about hair. From its types and what are the best ways to keep it healthy, strong and glamorous! This eBook will give you recipes and tips that are not only effective, but the ingredients can be found right in your kitchen! The things that you will find here are:

- Hair types, particularities according to individual types and how each one can be taken care of.
- Homemade recipes for all kinds of hair products.
- Some tips and tricks to make your hair beautiful in a matter of days!
- How you can take care of your hair on a daily basis.

By the time you complete this eBook, you will not be able to sit in your chair, but will be hitting the kitchen to prepare as many recipes for your hair as you can. Just keep in mind that there are some recipes that need to be followed exactly as they are, otherwise they might not give the results you were hoping for!

So without further discussion, let us dive into the world of *Natural Homemade Recipes for Long Healthy Hair* and how they are now in your hands!

Contents

Disclaimer 2

How This eBook is Just for Your Hair! 3

Introduction 9

Hair Types 101 10

    Important Thought 11

    Straight 11

    Curly 12

    Wavy 12

    Oily 12

    Normal 13

    Dry 13

    Combination Hair 13

    Small Tip 14

    Hair Color and How it Matters 15

        Blond 15

        Brunette 15

        Black 16

        Red 16

Recipes for Long, Healthy Tresses 17

Recipes for Oily Hair 18

   Growth Oils 18

   Nourishing Oil 18

   Body Adding Oil Treatment 19

   Jojoba & Lemon Oil Treatment 19

   Homemade Shampoos 21

   Rosemary and Peppermint Tea Shampoo 21

   Tea Tree Clarifying Shampoo 22

   Avocado Shampoo 22

   Organic Conditioners 24

   Herb Conditioner 24

   Honeyed Banana Conditioner 25

   Horsetail Conditioner 25

   Natural Hair Masks 27

   Curry Leaves in Coconut Oil 27

   Yogurt Mask 27

   Figs in Almond Oil 28

Recipes for Normal Hair 29

   Growth Oils 29

   Fresh Herb Oil 29

Rosemary Hot Oil 29

Burdock and Rosemary Oil 30

Homemade Shampoos 31

Refreshing Citrus and Cucumber Shampoo 31

Castile Soap Shampoo 31

Organic Cornstarch Shampoo 32

Organic Conditioners 33

Invigorating Coconut Milk Conditioner 33

Organic Shea Butter Conditioner 33

Avocado Hair Conditioner for Unmanageable Hair 34

Natural Hair Masks 35

Citrus Strawberry Hair Mask 35

Raw Egg Hair Mask 35

Creamy Oatmeal Hair Mask 36

Recipes for Dry Hair 37

Growth Oils 37

Ginger For Dry Hair Oil treatment 37

Organic sunflower and Lavender Oil 37

Castor oil growth oil 38

Homemade Shampoos 39

The Simply Organic Array Shampoo 39

Homemade Nettle Shampoo 39

Baking Soda Shampoo 40

Organic Conditioners 41

Mayo and Raw Egg Conditioner.. 41

Cider Vinegar Conditioner... 41

The Amplified Conditioner.. 42

Natural Hair Masks.. 43

Anti- Oxidant Rich Banana Hair Mask... 43

Olive Oil and Avocado Hair Mask... 44

Cinnamon Hair Mask.. 44

Facts and DIY Tips for Glorious Hair.. 46

The Balanced Diet 46

Flat Iron Blues.. 49

The Perfect Hair.. 50

Introduction

Beautiful, long, shiny hair has been a sign of beauty and health for women since forever and in all societies and cultures. Those who don't have it yearn for it, and those who do are always worried about losing it. Most times when women are not able to maintain healthy tresses a simple reason is that they don't take care of them. Keep in mind there is a difference between having healthy hair and fine hair. Just because you have fine hair doesn't mean they can't be healthy and beautiful.

Don't know much about hair types and how you need to take care of them? Aren't sure which category you fall in? Here is all the information you can possibly need.

Hair Types 101

The very first thing that you need to understand is that all hair is different. Just because a particular shampoo works for your sister does not mean it will give great results for your hair too. So ultimately you need to know your hair type to make sure that it is managed in the way required.

Dividing hair in different types is difficult, because there is oil and dry hair, fine and thick hair, curly and straight hair, blond, and brown hair and so much more. This eBook will tell you the basics of how you can distinguish what type of hair you have and what is the best way to make them long, strong and lustrous. Decide which type of hair you have and follow the recipes given below to achieve optimum results.

Important Thought

One idea that you need to remember is that healthy hair is not just a sign of beauty. It has been created for a purpose other than just to make you look beautiful. According to scientific fact, healthy people are bound to have healthy hair. Their function varies from providing warmth to protecting your head and giving an enhanced sense of touch. You can do without the presence of hair, but you will lose the various benefits that nature has blessed you with.

Once you understand the necessity of having beautifully healthy hair, making efforts to keep it that way becomes a lot easier. Here is some basic information about different varieties of hair.

Straight

As much as this can be the cause of envy among women who have wavy or curly hair, straight hair can be very difficult to manage. Yes the look is beautiful, but it also needs a lot of styling, just the right cut and shampooing every day. Compared to other hair kinds, straight hair tends to be finer, thinner and silkier. Since it is fine and thin, straight hair is mostly either oily or normal, depending on the type of skin you have.

Straight, fine hair is also more prone to hair loss and breakage. This is because it lacks in protein and is not as strong as it needs to be. But this too varies with individuals and cannot be generalized. Straight hair is considered to be a sign of elegance and sophistication.

Curly

Curly hair tends to be coarser, dryer and rough. This is because the hair cuticle and hair fiber is uneven. It can also be springy and thicker than straight, fine hair. There are many kinds of curls from loose big curls to tight and springy curls. Curly hair can also become very frizzy and uncontrollable if touched constantly, especially in winter months.

If you know how to manage it properly, then there is no hair type prettier than this. They always look full and give a sense of youth and vitality. While it might be rather difficult to grow; if taken care of properly can also become long and shiny.

Wavy

Wavy hair is the one that lies somewhere between straight and curly hair. By far the easiest to manage, wavy hair is neither too oily nor too dry. It can be grown long with relative ease as long as you feed it the right things. Since they are neither curly nor straight, this tress can make your hair look fuller and thicker. It adds a certain bounce to the hair and as long as you know how to take care of it, keeping them beautiful will not be a tough task for you.

Oily

Oily hair, just like oily skin can be a blessing and it can be a curse. It is great because you don't have a lot of trouble in winters. Usually it is naturally fine and most straight, so you can do without too much styling and as a bonus it doesn't fall as much as dry hair. Likewise oily hair is less prone to split ends.

But oily hair needs to be shampooed everyday if you don't want to go out in public with a head filled with greasy, dull looking hair. The reason why you might have oily hair is because the sebaceous glands on your scalp are very active. This means they provide more oil than needed and ends up making your hair look greasy. Oily hair also have more dandruff problems.

Normal

Normal hair is the best and most easily managed hair type. It isn't oily nor is it greasy. You can do away with washing normal hair for 3 or 4 days and not look it. It is also easy to style and can be shaped into however you like it. But it is still important to take proper care if you want lustrous and long hair.

Dry

Considered to be one of the most difficult hair types to manage, dry hair is the one most prone to breakage and gives a sense of lifelessness. The reason your hair is dry and brittle is that it lacks the ability to absorb and retain moisture. Also your sebaceous gland is not active and does not produce enough oil to keep the hair healthy and strong. The problem is thought to be genetic. It can be controlled and treated, but it cannot be reversed. Lack of vitamins and nutrients can also lead to hair dryness, as well as the excessive use of heat applications.

Combination Hair

Combination hair is a pain for those who have them. Combination hair type is one where the scalp is oily, yet the ends of hair are dry. This means that the hair is susceptible to breakage, hair loss, split ends and just about every other thing. But if you know the right ways to manage combination hair, it can also be kept healthy and beautiful.

People with curly or frizzy hair are the ones who mostly have combination hair.

Small Tip

There are many times when it isn't apparent whether you have dry, oily or normal hair. If you too aren't sure what your hair type is then try this simple test to be absolutely sure. Just take a tissue paper and press it in the center of the head, as well as both sides behind your ears. If the tissue paper has oil on it then it means you have oily hair but if the paper is dry then your hair type is dry. Normal hair is when your hair appears shiny without any oil in the center of your head. Combination hair is when you have oil in your scalp but dry looking hair at the end.

Once you have determined what kind of hair you have, taking care of the type becomes easier and more effective.

Hair Color and How it Matters

The color of your hair also makes a difference when it comes to caring for it. The color of your hair decides whether or not you should use some particular ingredients. Also hair color can make you look very different. Of course there are also various stereotypes associated with various hair colors! So here is some information for you.

Blond

The most common hair color among Northern and Eastern Europeans, natural blond color among adults can be found only among 2% of the population. It occurs because of a recessive mutation. Blond hair is often fine and thin.

There are various shades of blond hair colors ranging from pearly white blond to golden blond, strawberry blond to brownish blond. Many women opt to color their hair blond or get blond highlights in brown hair.

Blonds have been stigmatized with low IQ even though that is not true. They are susceptible to melanoma and an eye problem that can lead to blindness, known as age-related macular degeneration (AMD). So blondes need to be careful about such diseases.

Brunette

The second most common hair color, brown hair can mostly be found among people from West Eurasia, North America, Central Europe, Southern Europe and West Asia.

Brunette refers to both brown and black haired people, but completely black hair is listed as a separate hair color. The texture of brown hair can range from fine to coarse, moderately thick to thin. The color ranges from very dark brown to medium brown, chestnut to light brown hair.

Brunettes are thought to be the most reliable and loyal people. But they are also the ones who experience the most hair loss problems.

Black

The most common hair color, it occurs among 80% of the world population. It occurs among people of all ethnicities and countries. The shiniest kind of hair, if you have been blessed with this kind of hair, you might not need too many products to keep hair glowing all the time. The color black ranges from soft-black to jet black and even blue black.

Red

Considered to be the least commonly occurring hair color, red shade occurs because of the high consistency of pheomelanin in the hair. It is found in only 1-2% of people in the world and is mostly prominent in regions of Scotland and Ireland. The red color ranges from light strawberry blond to copper, titan and sometimes a flaming orangey red. True red color is very rare.

Redheads are considered to be fiery tempered and very passionate. They are also more prone to developing Parkinson's disease.

Recipes for Long, Healthy Tresses

Healthy hair, as mentioned above, is not just a sign of beauty, it is also a sign of good health. The problem of hair loss, dry and split ends has increased overtime because of the fact that women are becoming more and more dependent on chemical substances rather than natural, organic ingredients. These chemicals instead of improving the hair condition, only further aggravate the problem.

It is high time that both men and women go back in times and start opting for products that are manufactured through natural ingredients instead of relying on commercially constructed artificial hair care products. The recipes given below are not only simple to make and use, they are also as healthy as nature. You will only have to travel as far as your kitchen to find almost all the things required to care for your hair. Just make sure you follow the recipes accurately and keep using them over time. Some might not give results immediately and may need to be used for at least a month to show improvement.

Another small piece of advice is to use the recipe on one part of your scalp check its effects and if no reaction or allergy occurs, then start using it properly. Try to incorporate these recipes in your daily hair care routine and within no time your hair will be healthy and long!

Recipes for Oily Hair

Many women today are not very happy at the idea of oiling their hair. What they fail to understand is the basic rule, if you don't provide adequate nourishment to your scalp, your hair will never grow strong and long.

The idea of using oil on greasy hair may sound ridiculous but it actually works really well. Use of the right oil can make your hair lustrous and shiny before you have time to say 'Wow'! So oil your hair regularly, get rid of expensive, ineffective shampoos and say goodbye to conditioners that are made entirely of harmful chemicals. Here are some wonderful recipes for your oily hair.

Growth Oils

Almond oil, castor oil, coconut oil, olive oil, avocado oil and jojoba oil are said to be wonder oils when it comes to hair growth. Below are some recipes you can try and see which works best for you.

Nourishing Oil

Ingredients

2 tbsp olive oil

1 tbsp coconut oil

1 tbsp honey

1 tsp sea salt or Epsom salt

Process

Whisk all the ingredients together and heat it a little. Mix again and apply to slightly wet hair. Massage for 5 minutes. Soak a towel in hot water and squeeze out all the water. Cover your head with the towel and leave on for about 30-45 minutes. Rinse out with warm water and shampoo. Let dry naturally and brush your hair out.

Repeat the process at least once a week.

Body Adding Oil Treatment

Ingredients

4 tbsp sunflower oil

4 tbsp flat beer

1 egg

Process

Take the beer out in a glass and let all the carbon evaporate. Then add the oil and beaten egg to it mix well and apply to slightly damp hair. Leave on for half an hour and rinse with water and shampoo. Don't use too much shampoo. You can use this every other week to see best results. This will help in strengthening your hair.

Jojoba & Lemon Oil Treatment

Ingredients

1 cup Jojoba Oil

10 drops of lemon essential oil

1 tsp baking soda

Process

Combine all the ingredients and store in a glass bottle. When you want to use, heat up some oil, apply to the scalp and massage for some minutes. Then leave in oil in your hair overnight. Wash off the next day and let dry naturally. Repeat the process at least once a week.

Homemade Shampoos

These homemade shampoos are mild, effective, inexpensive and most importantly, keep your hair healthy and make it beautiful. Keep in mind though that when you initially start using them, it will feel like they don't really clean your hair, but after a while you will notice that they work better than any other commercial shampoo.

Rosemary and Peppermint Tea Shampoo

Ingredients

2 peppermint teabags

2 ½ cups of water

5 tbsp ivory soap

1 tbsp dried rosemary springs

2 drops rosemary essential oil *optional*

Process

Take the ivory soap bar and grate it. You will need about 5 tbsp. the rest of it can be stored for later use. Mix this grated soap in water and heat it up in a pan. When the soap has melted completely, remove from heat and add the teabags in the soap water mixture. Also add the crushed rosemary springs and essential oil. Lid the pan and let steep for about 10-15 minutes. Mix and strain. When it has cooled down, store in a plastic bottle. Use it every alternate day and see the results within a month! You will notice that you hair has started thickening.

Tea Tree Clarifying Shampoo

Ingredients

1 cup distilled water

¼ cup Castile soap *try getting one that is made of olive oil*

2 tbsp tea tree oil

2 drops of peppermint essential oil

Process

Boil the water and add all the ingredients to it. Mix until well combined and store in a bottle. Use every other day. Tea tree is excellent for clarifying the scalp and leaving it oil free. It combines with peppermint and works great for hair growth.

Avocado Shampoo

Ingredients

1 cup distilled water

¼ cup Castile liquid soap

Avocado oil 1 tsp

½ a mashed avocado

Process

Boil the water and add all ingredients to it. Blend and let cool. Apply to hair whenever taking a bath. Avocado is not just great for skin it also works wonders for hair growth. You can keep the shampoo bottle in the fridge to make it last longer.

Organic Conditioners

Conditioners are said to make your hair shiny, springy and look healthy from afar. But the use of chemically ridden conditioners only gives a shine for some time and their long term use is one of the major reasons for hair loss. This does not mean you should stop conditioning your hair. All it implies is that you opt for natural, homemade conditioners that you can use without having to worry about any extensive damage.

Herb Conditioner

Ingredients

A quart jar

Some nettles

Some marshmallows

Few sticks of cinnamon

Some distilled water

5-6 drops of lavender essential oil

Half a quart jar of apple cider vinegar

Process

Take nettles and marshmallows in the amount that it takes to fill up half the quart jar. Add vinegar, cinnamon sticks and lid tightly. Then place in a warm area for about 3 weeks. Once the time is over, take out the jar, strain the vinegar and add lavender essential oil to it, mix and store in a bottle. When using, mix one part conditioner with four parts of water. Rinse your hair with this mixture after shampooing. Be sure to wash with water afterwards.

Honeyed Banana Conditioner

Ingredients

1 pureed banana

¼ cup honey

2 drops of your favorite essential oil

Process

Simply mix all the ingredients well, add some water to make the mixture runnier and apply to slightly damp hair. Leave on for about 20 minutes and then wash off with warm water. Be sure it all gets out of your hair. You will love the feel of healthy, silky hair.

Horsetail Conditioner

Ingredients

2 cups boiled water

2 ½ tsp dried horsetail

Process

Simply steep the dried horsetail in boiled water for 20 minutes. After you have shampooed your hair, rinse your hair with this mixture. Let it sit for 10 minutes and then rinse your hair with cool water. After repeated use, you will feel a visible difference in your hair growth.

Natural Hair Masks

Hair masks are the added cherry on your cake. They help make your hair strong and give it the energy and nutrition required for quick growth. But the key thing to remember is to keep using them regularly. You can't expect to use them once a month and see amazing results. So make them a part of your once a week hair care routine.

Curry Leaves in Coconut Oil

Ingredients

A handful of fresh curry leaves

1 cup coconut oil

Process

Mix the oil and leaves and cook until a black residue starts appearing. Harvest the black residue and apply it to your scalp and hair twice a week. This will not only help your hair grow fast, it will also keep it safe from graying.

Yogurt Mask

Ingredients

Half a cup of natural and fresh yogurt

1/3 cup pureed fresh strawberries

1 tsp apple cider vinegar

1 tsp honey

Process

Mix all the ingredients well and apply to hair. Massage it into your scalp and spread to the hair. Leave it on for 20 minutes and then wash off thoroughly with warm water.

Figs in Almond Oil

Ingredients

3-4 mashed figs

3 tbsp almond oil

Process

Mix the ingredients well and massage gently into your scalp and hair. Leave on for about half an hour and then wash off with shampoo. Almond oil is an excellent ingredient for hair growth and since it is light, it will not grease your hair. Make sure you use this mask every week.

Recipes for Normal Hair

Growth Oils

Fresh Herb Oil

Ingredients

1 Oz fresh herbs

2 Oz Olive oil

Process

Soak the herbs in the oil in an air tight glass jar. (You can substitute olive oil with any other good quality vegetable oil if you like). Leave the jar on a windowsill, preferably under direct sunlight, for a month. This oil works best in summer. After the 30 days use cheesecloth to sieve the herbs from the oil and let the liquid oil filter to a clean jar.

Rosemary Hot Oil

Ingredients

12 drops lavender oil

6 drops rosemary oil

½ cup Sunflower oil

Process

Combine all the ingredients together and heat the mixture a bit, before applying the mask to slightly dampened hair from the roots to the tips. Cover your hair with a shower cap and let it be for around 20 minutes. Rinse off the mask with shampoo.

Burdock and Rosemary Oil

Ingredients

2 teaspoons basil oil

2 teaspoons rosemary oil

2 teaspoons lavender oil

2 teaspoons Aloe Vera gel

2 teaspoons burdock oil

Process

Mix all the ingredients together in a jar and apply generously into your hair; start from the scalp and apply the entire length of your hair toward the tips. Leave it in for around 4 to 5 hours before shampooing and washing it off. Remember though that the longer you will let this oil soak in to your hair the better the results. Use this oil once a week for up to 4 weeks.

Homemade Shampoos

Refreshing Citrus and Cucumber Shampoo

Ingredients

1 lemon

1 cucumber

Process

Peel 1 lemon and 1 cucumber and toss them in a blender. Blend until you get a smooth paste. This is all you need in your shampoo, scrub in your hair really well, as you want the pulps and chunks all absorbed through your hair. Rinse off with warm water.

Castile Soap Shampoo

Ingredients

¼ cup water

½ Oz tea tree oil

1 Oz apple cider vinegar

1 Cup liquid organic castile soap

Process

Mix all the ingredients in a blender and mix until smooth. You can use a spray bottle to store this too. All that you have to do is spray a bit of shampoo in your hair and scrub followed by rinsing it with warm water.

Organic Cornstarch Shampoo

Ingredients

Cornstarch as required

½ Oz baking soda

1 cup water

Process

Mix the water and baking soda together and gradually keep on adding a bit of cornstarch until you reach the desired consistency (it needs to be thick). Apply on your hair as shampoo and wash it off with lukewarm water. Enjoy showing off hair that has more volume and thickness.

Organic Conditioners

Invigorating Coconut Milk Conditioner

Ingredients

1 Oz coconut oil

1 avocado

1 cup coconut milk

Process

Peel the avocado and scoop out the seed. Use a food processor to crush the avocado until its smooth, add the coconut oil and milk and turn the processor on until the mixture is smooth. Apply the mixture on to your hair from the roots and cover the length of your hair. Let it soak in for at least 15 minutes before washing it off with warm water.

Organic Shea Butter Conditioner

Ingredients

1 tablespoon lavender oil

1 teaspoon vitamin E oil

2 teaspoon Olive oil

1 1/3 cup Shea butter

Process

Heat the Shea butter in order to make it liquid. Add olive oil while the butter is still hot and let the combination rest for approximately 35 minutes. Remember you cannot let the butter set into its original form. After the 35 minutes, mix in the Vitamin E oil and Lavender fragrance oil. You should have a mousse like product. Store this shampoo in an air tight container.

Avocado Hair Conditioner for Unmanageable Hair

Ingredients

1 Oz heavy cream

1 Oz water

1 Oz olive oil

1 avocado, pitted

1 teaspoon lavender oil

Process

Mix all the ingredients in a bowl and lather the conditioner in your hair, from the roots to the tips. Let the mixture sink in for at least 20 minutes and then simply rinse with water.

Natural Hair Masks

Citrus Strawberry Hair Mask

Ingredients

8 Strawberries

½ Oz coconut Oil

½ Oz honey

Process

Blend all the ingredients together, you do not have to make it a fine and smooth paste, it is okay if it ends up slightly chunky. Lightly wet your hair a bit and lather this paste into it. Leave it for around 8 minutes so that the nutrients like Vitamin C can sink in. Rinse off the mask with warm water only. The Citrus Strawberry hair mask gives off a very appealing scent of strawberries in your hair so make sure this is your final rinse.

Raw Egg Hair Mask

Ingredients

1 raw egg

¾ cup milk

½ lemon, nicely squeezed

1 Oz olive oil

Process

Use only the egg yolks (separate the whites and yolks beforehand); whisk them first in a dry bowl and add the milk and olive oil once they are nicely beaten. Mix the ingredients well and add the few drops of lemon juice in the end.

Slather them thoroughly in your scalp and hair. Remember to use a shower cap and let your hair be for 15 minutes. Rinse with lukewarm water and make sure you get all the egg-y chunks out of your hair by combing through while you wash your hair. For a final rinse use an organic shampoo so that your head does not continue smelling like raw eggs.

Creamy Oatmeal Hair Mask

Ingredients

½ Oz Oats

½ Oz fresh milk

1/12 Oz almond oil

Process

Mix all the ingredients, you can use a food blender here. The result should be a thick paste. Because of its consistency, make sure that you have combed your hair through beforehand so that applying this mask becomes easier. Lather the mask well and thoroughly from the roots to the tips. You need to leave it in for a minimum duration of 20 minutes, after which you will have to rinse through with shampoo and hot water.

Recipes for Dry Hair

Growth Oils

Ginger For Dry Hair Oil treatment

Ingredients

1 teaspoon natural lemon juice

1 teaspoon sesame oil

1 ginger root

Process

It is preferable if you use organic oil. You will have to squeeze out the juice of the ginger root and make sure you collect around ½ an Oz of juice. Mix all the ingredients together and apply to the scalp and the length of your hair. Make sure the mixture dries before you rinse it off with warm water. This mask works best if you use it at least 3 times a week.

Organic sunflower and Lavender Oil

Ingredients

10 drops geranium oil

10 drops lavender oil

10 drops sandalwood

½ cup organic sunflower oil

Process

Leave the oil and mix the rest of the ingredients thoroughly. Heat the oil a bit, but don't make it scalding hot, and add that to the mask mixture. Damp your hair a bit and lather the mixture thoroughly from the roots to the tips. Cover your hair with a shower cap and let the mask sink in for around 20 minutes. Use an organic shampoo to rinse off the mask.

Castor oil growth oil

Ingredients

30 drops of Castor oil

20 drops of almond oil

Process

Mix the two oils together and apply to your hair thoroughly. Remember to cover your hair with a shower cap and allow thenutritive properties of the oil soak in overnight. Use this once a week every week for over a month.

Tip: you can use this oil mixed with conditioner to dilute its greasiness and apply it every other day.

Homemade Shampoos

The Simply Organic Array Shampoo

Ingredients

½ cup homemade coconut milk

2/3 Liquid Castile soap

1 teaspoon Vitamin E oil

30 drops of essential oils (whatever you prefer)

1 teaspoon almond oil

Process

Mix all ingredients in an air tight container or an old empty shampoo bottle. Shake the bottle to mix the contents. You will only need around a teaspoon when you are shampooing your hair with this.

Tip: You can let the ingredients rest in an airtight jar a month before using for better results.

Homemade Nettle Shampoo

Ingredients

100 ml castor oil

4 Vials Vitamin B complex

50 ml stinging nettle extract

1 Oz Panthenol solution

100 ml nettle shampoo, organic

Process

Mix all the materials and place in an air tight glass jar or container. You need to use this shampoo consistently for a couple of months for glorious hair results.

Baking Soda Shampoo

Ingredients

1 tablespoon baking soda

1 ½ cup water

Process

Combine the two ingredients and store it in an empty shampoo bottle. No need to let the mixture settle on its own for any duration of time.

Organic Conditioners

Mayo and Raw Egg Conditioner

Ingredients

1 raw egg

½ cup mayonnaise

½ cup yogurt

Process

Separate the egg yolk from the egg white and only use the whites. Beat all the ingredients together and apply to your hair thoroughly, make sure you lather an extra amount on the damaged strands. Cover your hair with a shower cap and leave the conditioner in for at least 25 minutes (it's a tedious conditioner but it works wonders). Remember to wash it off with lukewarm water. Hot water thickens the egg and you end up with itty bitty pieces of eggs tangled in your hair.

Cider Vinegar Conditioner

Ingredients

3 cups cold water

1 cup cider vinegar

Process

Mix the two ingredients and store them in a plastic bottle. After shampooing, apply thoroughly into your hair but do not rinse. The Cider Vinegar conditioner works as a leave in conditioner.

The Amplified Conditioner

Ingredients

Cider Vinegar conditioner (see above)

½ teaspoon water

1 tablespoon thick honey

5 tablespoons baking soda

Process

Combine all ingredients together except the water and when the mixture becomes thick and pasty, start adding a couple of drops of water as you keep mixing the conditioner. Store the mixture in an empty and unbreakable bottle. After shampooing, lather the conditioner into your hair all the way the length of it. Let the mixture and its constituent ingredients soak in for 5 minutes before you rinse it off.

Natural Hair Masks

Anti- Oxidant Rich Banana Hair Mask

Ingredients

1 tablespoon honey

½ Oz Olive oil

½ Oz coconut oil

2 Bananas

Process

It is more preferable if you choose bananas that have browned a bit over time. Blend the two bananas alone, until they become a smooth paste. This will take a couple of minutes more than regular blending. Toss in the oil, coconut and honey into this smooth mixture and blend to make a smoothie.

Rub this mixture into your scalp and lather it into your hair nicely. It will take 5 minutes for the nutrients to kick in so let the mixture sink in for that time at least. Rinse with warm water and while you are doing it, remember you should be combing through your hair too, so that none of it is left in. The best thing about this mask is that bananas smell really good and you do not need another final rinse to remove the fruity scent.

Olive Oil and Avocado Hair Mask

Ingredients

½ cup milk

½ Oz almond oil

1 small Avocado

Process

It is preferable that you choose a ripe avocado. Cut the avocado into small pieces and blend them until they are smooth. Toss the almond oil and milk into this smooth mixture and blend well. Lather the mask into the scalp and let it sink in while you apply to the length of your hair. Remember, for this mask you will need to wear a hair cap and wait for around 16 minutes before you rinse it out with warm water.

Cinnamon Hair Mask

Ingredients

5 Tablespoon Virgin Olive oil

2 eggs

1 tablespoon honey

2 tablespoon Cinnamon powder

Process

Mix all the ingredients together; you can whisk them, no need for a blender. Apply the mixture to your roots and slather thoroughly to the length of your hair. Let the mixture sink in for at least 14 minutes. For this hair mask you will have to rinse your hair with shampoo.

Facts and DIY Tips for Glorious Hair

The Balanced Diet

This entire eBook consists of natural ways to make your hair healthy and beautiful. You must keep in mind that your hair is a part of you, and your health affects the health of your hair too. In other words, using natural products and health benefitting products on your hair is all good, but there is another easier thing that you can do that will automatically work wonders for your hair.

Mount Up the Calories

Counting your calorie intake is the worst thing you could do to your hair. Sure, you are dying to get into those size 0 jeans but what is the point of it if you end up with a bunch of hay for hair.

Eating the right foods and enough food is sure to make your hair lively again as it needs its own sustenance.

Say No to Processed Food

Processed foods though highly convenient do not provide the necessary nutrients that the food name promises. The reason this is so is that processed food does not hesitate to destroy many of the essential elements in the processing method. Whole foods on the other hand are rich in them. The best thing about switching from processed foods to whole meals is that there is next to nothing of a difference in calories in both. The whole foods provide you with the vitamins and nutrients that your hair craves.

Protein Is The Secret Ingredient.

Don't go by what they say about there being no secret ingredient. I mean so many of us have to keep in shape and we cannot afford to start chowing down on everything tempting just to get thicker hair (and ultimately a wider belt). The only thing to do here would be to resort to a protein diet. And here is the good news: A protein rich diet can solely make the journey to longer and thicker tresses. Protein not only helps hair growth but aids in rejuvenating your skin and nails.

If you are ready to focus on a protein rich diet for your hair, look for victuals rich in alkaline elements, this will prevent collagen breakdown from acidic foods like dairy and poultry. Boost your protein intake from leafy greens, sunflower seeds, avocados, pumpkin seeds, flax, chia and hemp.

Caffeine Hates You

It is true and women are usually surprised by this. This means soda, coffee, black tea and energy drinks. Save for green tea, the caffeine in all these drinks are bad for your hair. The bottom line is that caffeine functions to eliminate the vital nutrients from existing in your body that help thicken your hair. If you cannot get rid of the habit of caffeine then start by switching to green tea in the time that you are used to having caffeine during the day. When you consume caffeine what experts dub as 'beauty minerals' (sulfur, B vitamins, magnesium and potassium) are excreted from your body through urine.

Omega 3

Consume Omega 3 and Omega 6 fats. They quicken the growth process of your hair by boosting the collagen reserves towards them. The side effects of that are good too as your skin will reduce blemishes and marks and your metabolism will get better. Food like fish, flax seeds and walnuts are rich in omega 3.

Pro Vitamin A

Also known popularly as beta carotene. Vitamin A works to repair hair and skin. They aid in thickening the hair and pump strength into it. The best sources of Vitamin A are spinach, sweet potato, cantaloupe, Swiss chard, kale, papaya, peaches, mango, tomatoes and peppers. The amazing part about Pro Vitamin A is that you only need to consume it for a very short time for it to show results. Plus it is known to easily permeate into your bloodstream.

Good Fats

Eating for the love of your hair is probably the best and easiest way in the book. There are tons of dietary tips just for the hair. Healthy fats do not come from sources like fast food. Victuals like walnuts, almonds, coconut, hemp, flax, chia, trout, tuna and salmon are great sources rich in good fats. Unlike other healthy foods, healthy fats boost the shine in your hair and increase the length of your hair.

If you make it a point to practice a balanced diet and not over eat food rich in good fats you would be availing the advantages all the while barring yourself from becoming fat.

Good fats start showing their results in around a month's time. Plus as a bonus, many sources of healthy fats have slimming effects too.

Flat Iron Blues

Even though you might use a numerous array of natural and organic products for the sake of your hair, let us not forget the number of times one runs to the aid of flat irons to style the mousy mess one thinks he or she sees on their head.

Flat irons are more popular than hair dryers today. It only made sense to add this in the contents of this eBook due to the much talked about problems in using a flat iron.

The Material of the Iron

The first thing that you must give your attention to is purchasing the right plates for the flat irons. Seriously, they have sapphire, titanium, ion, ceramic and tourmaline flat irons in the market. The wisest choice out of these would be ceramic as they use less heat and less time to completely penetrate the hair shaft. This will also reduce the UV damage to your hair as much as possible.

The next best choice would be to use tourmaline plates; they lower the frizz in your hair by creating negative ions and boost the pressure when heating the hair so that the hair ends up sleek and shiny.

Heat Protectants

Since the word of the day is natural remedies for your hair, you must acknowledge that heat protectants have no substitute. You must remember to dry your hair completely before dabbing this on it. Failure to apply heat protectant to your hair before flat ironing it can result in fried hair. A good tip is that you avoid applying the protectant near the roots of your hair as that act can make your hair look greasy.

Purchase the Iron with Heat Settings

A lot of flat irons have a built in custom thermostat. This however does not mean that the hotter you make the iron the better it would do to your hair. Usually the prime setting would be to set the iron on no more than 300. But if your hair is really thick you can easily go up to 380 too.

As much as any hair style tempts you, you must remember to take a break from treating your hair to scalding plates. Frequent users should remember to use moisturizing conditioners that will counteract the effects of the flat iron.

The Perfect Hair

As much as anyone thinks of the perfect tresses as a miracle at work. It is actually pretty easy. Organic and natural methods that produce shampoos and conditioners are evidently far less complex and more benefitting in their nutrient rich properties than the alkaline solutions we pay hefty sums for. If you look at it in a logical way and count the time you usually take to care for your hair when on a tight schedule; it hardly differs from that of what one would expect you to spend in convenient hair chemical products.

www.ingramcontent.com/pod-product-compliance
Lightning Source LLC
Chambersburg PA
CBHW052017280526
45793CB00005B/1013